REVISED EDITION

VITAMINS

HERBS, MINERALS & SUPPLEMENTS

THE COMPLETE GUIDE

REVISED EDITION

VITAMINS

HERBS, MINERALS & SUPPLEMENTS

THE COMPLETE GUIDE

H. WINTER GRIFFITH, M.D.

Technical Consultant

Cynthia Thomson, M.S., R.D.

Clinical Nutrition Research Specialist, Arizona Cancer Center
University of Arizona Prevention Center

Da Capo
LIFE
LONG

A Member of the Perseus Books Group

Library of Congress Cataloging-in-Publication available from the Library of Congress

ISBN-13: 978-1-55561-263-4
ISBN-10:1-55561-263-6

Cover Photo: Larry Williams/Masterfile
Cover: Gary D. Smith, Performance Design

Da Capo Press is a member of the Perseus Books Group.
www.dacapopress.com

Da Capo Press books are available at special discounts for bulk purchases in the U.S. by corporations, institutions, and other organizations. For more information, please contact the Special Markets Department at the Perseus Books Group, 11 Cambridge Center, Cambridge MA 02142, or call (800) 255-1514 or email special.markets@perseusbooks.com

15 16 17 18 19 20 21 22 23 24 - 07 08 09

Contents

About the Author

H. Winter Griffith, M.D., received his medical degree from Emory University in 1953 and spent more than 20 years in private practice. At Florida State University, he established a basic medical science program and also directed the family practice residency program at Tallahassee Memorial Hospital. After moving to the Southwest, he became associate professor of Family and Community Medicine at the University of Arizona College of Medicine. He devoted most of his time to writing medical-information books for general readers.

Dedication

To each of you who wishes to be informed enough to become the most important member of your own healthcare team.

Acknowledgments

Several years ago, Dr. Griffith set a personal goal to translate complicated, technical medical information into easy-to-understand terms that anyone outside the healing professions could use. Four previous books dealing with medications, symptoms, surgery and sports injuries have been major steps toward that goal.

Dr. Griffith remained a student of medicine for 40 years. The need for this book was made clear during his experience as a family doctor, teacher and author, answering questions (or seeking answers) for patients, medical students, nurses and physicians in training.

Special thanks to Sheldon Saul Hendler, M.D., Ph.D., author of *The Complete Guide to the Anti-Aging Nutrients* (Simon & Schuster, 1984; Fireside, 1986) for allowing the use of his material and unique research insights in this book.

Thanks also to everyone else who helped with this book in so many ways, including Brian Engstrom and Jean Anderson, research assistants, and technical consultant Cynthia Thomson, M.S., R.D., who is a registered dietitian with more than 18 years of clinical experience in nutrition. She is currently completing her Ph.D. in Nutritional Sciences at the University of Arizona, where she also works as an investigator on nutritional breast-cancer research trials. She facilitates the Nutritional Medicine Core for the Department of Medicine's program in Integrative Medicine, the first such training program in the United States.

Last but not least, thanks to the authors and publishers of the reference material (listed in the Bibliography) that was so helpful in the preparation of this book.

Vitamins and Minerals

Surveys show that more than half of the U.S. adult population uses dietary supplements of one type or another. In 1996 alone, consumers spent more than $6.5 billion on dietary supplements, according to one New York market-research firm. But even with all the purchases they generate, consumers still ask questions about dietary supplements: Can their claims be trusted? Are they safe? Does the Food and Drug Administration (FDA) approve them?

Many of these questions come in the wake of the 1994 Dietary Supplement Health and Education Act (DSHEA). The Act set up a new framework for FDA regulation of dietary supplements. This legislation created a new office within the National Institutes of Health to coordinate research on dietary supplements, called the Office of Alternative Medicine (OAM). It also provided for an independent dietary-supplements commission to report on the use of claims in dietary-supplement labeling.

The Council for Responsible Nutrition, an organization of manufacturers of dietary supplements and their suppliers, welcomes the change. "Our philosophy has been to maintain consumer access to products and access to information so that consumers can make informed choices," says John Cordaro, the group's president and chief executive officer.

Although the FDA receives numerous questions from consumers, who want to know whether they should use dietary supplements, the agency so far is limited in its ability to respond. Under the provisions of DSHEA, the FDA works under less rigid guidelines for pre-market review of dietary supplements than it does for other products it regulates, such as drugs and many additives used in processed foods. This means consumers and manufacturers, *not* the government, are responsible for checking the safety of dietary supplements and determining the truthfulness of label claims.

Effective in March 1999, the following information must appear on the labels of dietary supplements:

- Statement of identity (for example, "ginseng")
- Net quantity of contents (for example, "60 capsules")

- Structure-function claim *and* the message, "This statement has not been evaluated by the Food and Drug Administration. This product is not intended to diagnose, treat, cure or prevent any disease." (A structure-function claim refers to the purpose of or benefit derived from using the product.)
- Directions for use (for example, "Take one capsule daily.")
- Supplement Facts Panel (lists serving size, amount and active ingredient)
- Other ingredients in descending order of predominance and by common name or proprietary blend
- Name and place of business of manufacturer, packer or distributor. This is the address to which to write for more product information

In addition, the American Institute of Nutrition and the American Society for Clinical Nutrition have issued an official statement on vitamin and mineral supplements. This statement was developed jointly with the American Dietetic Association and the National Council against Health Fraud. The American Medical Association's Council on Scientific Affairs reviewed the statement and found it to be consistent with its official statement on dietary supplements.

The statement reads: "Healthy children and adults should obtain adequate nutrient intakes from dietary sources. Meeting nutrient needs by choosing a variety of foods in moderation, rather than by supplementation, reduces the potential risk for both nutrient deficiencies and nutrient excesses. Individual recommendations regarding supplements and diets should come from physicians and registered dietitians."

Supplementation is sometimes necessary in various circumstances. Some of these situations are listed below.

- Women with excessive menstrual bleeding may need iron supplements.
- Pregnant or breastfeeding women have an increased need for certain nutrients, especially iron, folic acid and calcium.
- People with very low calorie intakes frequently consume diets that do not meet their needs for most nutrients.
- Some vegetarians may not receive adequate calcium, iron, zinc and vitamin B-12.
- Newborns are commonly given a single dose of vitamin K to prevent abnormal bleeding. (This is done under the direction of a physician.)
- Certain disorders or diseases and some medications interfere with nutrient intake, digestion, absorption, metabolism or excretion. In addition, expanding scientific research indicates that supplementation with specific nutrients may be beneficial in the prevention of disease. Those who suffer myocardial infarction, for example, may benefit from vitamin-E supplementation.

Nutrients are potentially toxic when ingested in sufficiently large amounts. Safe intake levels vary widely from nutrient to nutrient and may vary with an individual's age and health. In addition, high-dosage vitamin and mineral supplements can interfere with the normal metabolism of other nutrients and with the therapeutic effects of certain drugs. The Recommended Dietary Allowance (RDA) and the Dietary Reference Intake (DRI) represent the best currently available assessments of safe and adequate intakes. They serve as the basis for the Recommended Daily Allowances shown on many product labels, although these are determined by the FDA for labeling purposes and should not be used by individuals as guidelines for their own daily intake. *Recommended Daily Allowances are not the same as Recommended Dietary Allowances.*

Every health professional wants consumers to take proper nutrients and supplements if they need them, but some people abuse these essential substances by taking doses 10 to 20 times the recommended amount or more.

Some people believe if one pill is good, 20 pills must be better. They also believe vitamins, minerals, herbs and supplements are medicine.

As information in this book points out, vitamins, minerals, herbs and supplements can cause side effects, adverse reactions, and interactions with other drugs and nutrients. Many individuals need to avoid certain substances because of a unique situation, such as pregnancy or age. Others need to be aware that medical conditions, such as heart problems or various disease conditions, can be an indication not to take certain substances.

When deciding whether or not to supplement your diet with vitamins and minerals, remember that too much can be harmful. For example, high doses of vitamin A can cause bone pain and vomiting. High doses of vitamin C can also have toxic effects, including diarrhea and perhaps kidney stones. Too much of this vitamin can interfere with white blood cells' ability to kill bacteria. This can make infections worse rather than clear them up.

Many conditions may also rule out taking some substances. Always be alert to any side effects or interactions you may experience that could put your health in jeopardy. It's up to you to be a "smart" consumer of the vitamins, minerals and supplements your body may need. Get them from the food you eat when you can—supplement with available products when you must.

Vitamins

Vitamins are chemical compounds necessary for growth, health, normal metabolism and physical well-being. Some vitamins are essential parts of *enzymes*—the chemical molecules that catalyze or facilitate the completion of chemical reactions. Other vitamins form essential parts of *hormones*— the chemical substances that promote and protect body health and reproduction. If you're in good health, you need vitamins only in small amounts. They can be found in sufficient quantities in the foods you eat. This assumes you eat a normal, well-balanced diet of foods grown in nutritionally adequate soil.

Traditionally, vitamins have been divided into two categories: *fat-soluble* and *water-soluble.*

Fat-soluble vitamins can be stored in the body. If you take excessive amounts of fat-soluble vitamins, they accumulate to provide needed amounts at a later time. That's the good news. The bad news is, if you take excessive amounts of fat-soluble vitamins, toxic levels can accumulate in storage areas such as the liver. Too much of any fat-soluble vitamin can lead to potentially dangerous, long-term physical problems.

Water-soluble vitamins cannot be stored in the body to any great extent. The daily amount you need must be provided by what you eat over several days.

The amount of vitamins you need increases during illness, following surgery or even as a result of the aging process. In these circumstances, vitamin supplements may be necessary to meet increased needs or prevent a deficiency of select nutrients.

People with special needs for supplements or others at risk of vitamin deficiency are identified and discussed in detail later in this section. See page 10.

Vitamin supplements cannot take the place of good nutrition. Vitamins do not provide energy. Your body needs other substances besides vitamins for adequate nutrition, including carbohydrates, fats, proteins and minerals. Vitamins cannot help maintain a healthy body except in the presence of other nutrients, mainly from food and minerals.

Minerals

Minerals are inorganic chemical elements. They participate in many biochemical and physiological processes necessary for optimum growth, development and health. There is a clear and important distinction between the terms *mineral* and *trace element.* If the body requires more than 100 milligrams of a mineral each day, the substance is labeled *mineral.* If the body requires less than 100 milligrams of a mineral each day, the substance is labeled *trace element.*

Many minerals are essential parts of enzymes. They also participate actively in regulating many physiological functions, including transporting oxygen to each of the body's 60 trillion cells, providing the stimulus for muscles to contract and in many ways guaranteeing normal function of the central nervous system. Minerals are required for growth, maintenance, repair and health of tissues and bones.

Most minerals are widely distributed in foods. *Severe* mineral deficiency is unusual in the Western world. Of all essential minerals, only a few may be deficient in a typical diet. Iron deficiency can be seen in infants, children and pregnant women. Zinc and copper deficiencies are also not uncommon, especially during illness.

Multivitamin/Mineral Preparations

A varied diet will contain all the nutrients you need. For healthy people food is the best, most reliable source of nutrients. If you or your children need supplementation, the best place to start is by taking one of the commercially available multivitamin/mineral preparations. Commercial over-the-counter products usually have a good balance of nutrients. Taking separate products can lead to an imbalance of nutrients, which can lead to an overabundance of one substance at the expense of decreased absorption or effectiveness of another.

Taking separate, individual nutrient supplements will require careful consideration of nutrient-to-nutrient interactions and is more likely to result in excess intake above what may be healthy—in these cases you may want to talk with your doctor, dietitian or pharmacist. The cost tends to be lower if you take a combination product rather than separate products.

Most major pharmaceutical manufacturers supply widely advertised combination products. The brand names are too numerous to list and they change constantly. Your pharmacist, doctor or dietitian should be able to recommend a good source for a superior multivitamin/mineral preparation.

If you study vitamins and minerals, you may find you need supplements for one reason or another. We hope this book provides you with enough information to choose wisely or be able to ask the right questions to find out what is best for you.

Guide to Vitamin, Mineral and Acid Charts

Information in this book is organized in condensed, easy-to-read charts, divided into five main sections: vitamins, minerals, amino acids and nucleic acids, other supplements and medicinal herbs. (Information on the supplement and medicinal-herb sections and charts begins on page 20.) Each substance is described in a multipage format as shown in the sample charts on the following pages. They are arranged alphabetically by the most frequently recognized name—usually a generic name instead of a brand name.

The most common names of substances appear at the top of the chart. For example, vitamin C is frequently called *ascorbic acid.* Both names appear at the top of the chart. Less common names are listed in the first section of the chart, *Basic Information.*

To learn more about any vitamin or mineral, you need to know only one name. Look in the Index for any name you know, page 497. The Index provides a page number for the information you seek about that substance.

The next few pages provide an explanation for each section of a vitamin, mineral, or acid

chart. The numbers correspond to the sample chart on pages 8 and 9. This information will help you read and understand the charts that begin on page 28.

1–Generic name

Each chart is titled by the *generic name,* the official chemical name of the substance. If two or more generic names exist, the substance is alphabetized by the most common name, with other names in parentheses at the top of the page or listed under the *Basic Information* section. If a substance has two or more generic names, the Index includes a reference for each name.

A product container may show a generic name, a brand name or both. If the container has no name, ask the pharmacist or health-store attendant for the name.

2–Available from natural sources?

3–Available from synthetic sources?

Many vitamins, minerals and supplements are advertised as

"natural," implying the product is derived from natural sources as opposed to synthetic sources. By definition, minerals are basic chemical substances that can't be manufactured (or synthesized) from other substances. However, many vitamins and supplements are derived from both natural and synthetic sources.

This is confusing to many consumers. Many manufacturers have done everything possible to take financial advantage of that confusion. Advertisers claim natural sources are good and synthetic sources are bad. The truth is, natural and synthetic versions of the same chemical are identical!

Don't pay extra money for *natural* vitamins or supplements. They all have the same effect on your body. The *synthetic* version may be even purer or less contaminated with extraneous materials such as insecticides and fertilizers.

4—Prescription required?

Most vitamins, minerals and supplements are available without prescription. Some formulas with higher dosages to treat specific diseases require a prescription from your doctor. "Yes" means your doctor must prescribe. "No" means you can buy this product without prescription. "Yes, for some" means that certain dosages or forms (such as an injection) require a prescription while others do not.

The information about a generic product is the same, whether it requires a prescription or not. If the generic ingredients are the same, nonprescription products have the same uses, dangers, warnings, precautions, side effects and interactions with other substances that prescription products do.

5—Fat-soluble or water-soluble?

This line applies *only* to vitamins. Fat-soluble vitamins can accumulate in the body and might cause toxic effects in excessive doses, either in a single day or in small, periodic excesses over a long time. Water-soluble vitamins do not accumulate to any great extent in the body. Except under unusual circumstances, the body readily eliminates excess water-soluble accumulation. The dangers of water-soluble vitamins generally depend on the effects of excessive dosages taken over a relatively short period.

6—RDA/DRI and Optimal Intake

This line points you to the page where you'll find information about the substance's Recommended Dietary Allowance (RDA), Dietary Reference Intake (DRI), and Optimal Intake whenever this information is available. Not all substances will have this information for a few possible reasons: Some substances are still under study;

Guide to Vitamin, Mineral and Acid Charts

To find information about a specific vitamin, mineral, or acid, look in the easy-to-read charts starting on page 28. Charts like the sample shown below and on the opposite page appear alphabetically by generic name.

38   BIOTIN

1 — ## Biotin (Vitamin H)

Basic Information

2 — • Available from natural sources? Yes
3 — • Available from synthetic sources? No
4 — • Prescription required? No
5 — • Water-soluble
6 — • *RDA/DRI and Optimal Intake,* see page XXX

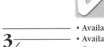

7 — ### Natural Sources

Almonds	Liver
Bananas	Mackerel
Brewer's yeast	Meats
Brown rice	Milk
Bulgur wheat	Mushrooms
Butter	Oat bran
Calf liver	Oatmeal
Cashew nuts	Peanut butter
Cheese	Peanuts
Chicken	Salmon
Clams	Soybeans
Eggs, cooked	Split peas
Green peas	Tuna
Lentils	Walnuts

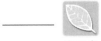

8 — ### Benefits

• Aids formation of fatty acids
• Facilitates metabolism of amino acids and carbohydrates
• Promotes normal health of sweat glands, nerve tissue, bone marrow, male sex glands, blood cells, skin, hair
• Minimizes symptoms of zinc deficiency

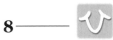

9 — ### Possible Additional Benefits

• May alleviate muscle pain
• May alleviate depression

Who May Benefit from Additional Amounts? — **10**

People who consume huge quantities of raw eggs, which contain a compound (avidin) that inhibits biotin. (Cooking eggs destroys this compound and eliminates the problem.)

Deficiency Symptoms — **11**

Note: Deficiency is extremely rare.

Babies:
• Dry scaling on scalp and face

Adults:
• Fatigue
• Depression
• Nausea
• Loss of appetite
• Loss of muscular reflexes
• Smooth, pale tongue
• Hair loss
• Increased blood-cholesterol levels
• Anemia
• Conjunctivitis
• Liver enlargement

Usage Information

What this vitamin does: — **12**
Biotin is necessary for normal growth, development and health.

Miscellaneous information: — **13**
Intestinal bacteria produce all the biotin the body needs, so there is no substantial evidence that normal, healthy adults need dietary supplements of biotin.

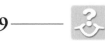

14— **Available as:**
• Tablets or capsules: Swallow whole with a full glass of liquid. Don't chew or crush. Take with food or immediately after eating to decrease stomach irritation.
• Biotin is a constituent of many multivitamin/mineral preparations.

 Warnings and Precautions

15— **Don't take if you:**
No problems are expected.

16— **Consult your doctor if you:**
No problems are expected.

17— **Over 55:**
No problems are expected.

18— **Pregnancy:**
• No problems are expected.
• Don't take doses greater than DRI.

19— **Breastfeeding:**
• No problems are expected.
• Don't take doses greater than DRI.

20— **Effect on lab tests:**
No expected effects.

21— **Storage:**
• Store in a cool, dry place away from direct light, but don't freeze.
• Store safely out of reach of children.
• Don't store in bathroom medicine cabinet. Heat and moisture may change the action of the vitamin.

 Overdose/Toxicity

22— **Signs and symptoms:**
Supplements in amounts suggested by manufacturers on the label are nontoxic.

What to do: ————————— **—23**
For accidental overdose (such as child taking entire bottle): Dial 911 (emergency), 0 for operator or call your nearest Poison Control Center.

Adverse Reactions or Side Effects **—24**
None are expected if taken within DRI dosage levels.

Interaction with Medicine, Vitamins or Minerals **—25**

Interacts with	Combined effect
Long term antibiotics (broad spectrum)	Destroys "friendly" bacteria in intestines that produce biotin. This can lead to significant biotin deficiency.
Sulfonamides	Destroys "friendly" bacteria in intestines that produce biotin. This can lead to significant biotin deficiency.

Interaction with Other Substances **—26**
Tobacco decreases absorption. Smokers may require supplemental biotin.

Alcohol decreases absorption.

Foods:
Eating large quantities of raw egg whites may cause biotin deficiency. Egg whites contain avidin, which prevents biotin from being absorbed into the body.

Lab Tests to Detect Deficiency **—27**
None are available, except for experimental purposes.

VITAMINS

some substances are abundantly available in food, so deficiency and excess are rare to non-existent and no guidelines are necessary; some substances are so rare, no guidelines have been established.

7–Natural Sources

This section lists the food and beverage sources from which vitamins, minerals and acids may be obtained. They are listed alphabetically, not in order of the richest sources of the substance. If you want more information about natural sources, many reference works are available at your local library.

8–Benefits

This section consists of *proved benefits*, including body functions the substance maintains or improves. It also lists disease processes and malfunctions the substance cures or improves. These proved benefits have withstood the scrutiny of scientifically controlled studies with results published in medical literature. This medical literature is subjected to review by top authorities in many fields before the material can be published in respected scientific journals.

9–Possible Additional Benefits

Some authors and many newspaper, magazine and television advertisers make unjustified, sometimes outrageous, claims for products. This list contains claims that have *not* withstood the same scientific scrutiny the *Benefits* section has passed. These claims may be as accurate and as effective as the proven claims, but they haven't been proved with well-controlled studies. Such studies can take years to complete and may be very expensive. Until such studies have been completed, the claims must be listed as possible additional benefits. Do not self-medicate based on these unproven benefits!

10–Who May Benefit from Additional Amounts?

People listed in this category are most likely to need significant care to regain or maintain normal health or are less likely to meet their requirements through diet alone. A summary of groups follows, with a list of reasons why the risk is greater.

Anyone with inadequate dietary intake or increased nutritional needs—Included in this group are people whose energy needs are less than 1,200 calories a day. Fewer than 1,200 calories a day for energy requirements almost never provides enough vitamins and minerals, so supplements are needed. Those most likely to have inadequate dietary intake include

- People of small stature or build who eat only minimal nutrients per day to maintain current weight
- Elderly people with greatly decreased daily activities, particularly aging women

- People who have had limbs amputated
- People with reduced physical activity because of activity-limiting disease, such as coronary-artery disease, intermittent lameness, angina pectoris
- Fad dieters with a dietary imbalance and inadequacy
- People with eating disorders such as anorexia nervosa or bulimia
- Vegetarians

People over 55—People in this age group may have inadequate dietary intake because of difficulty obtaining an adequate diet, or because of disability and depression.

Pregnancy—Pregnant women uniformly need supplementation of folic acid and iron. Sometimes they need other supplements as well. Pregnant women need to increase dietary intake so total body weight increases from 12 to 30 pounds during pregnancy. Many women do not consume enough calories to allow this weight gain and therefore develop a nutritional deficiency. This causes a need for supplementation with a well-rounded, well-balanced preparation containing vitamins and minerals in addition to separate supplementation of folic acid and iron.

Ask your doctor to recommend specific brand names of acceptable multivitamin/mineral preparations. Also seek advice about folic acid and iron.

Breastfeeding women—Breastfeeding women who are healthy

and active may need to continue supplementation, especially iron. Consult your doctor.

Most authorities suggest that iron and folic-acid supplements for pregnant and breastfeeding women should be taken as separate products. Iron occasionally causes gastrointestinal side effects that are so uncomfortable to some women that they discontinue the supplements.

Another important nutritional factor with breastfeeding is the need for extra fluids. Fluid deficiency can be as disabling as a nutritional deficiency. Drink at least eight 8-ounce glasses of water a day.

People who abuse alcohol and other drugs—People who consume too much alcohol are likely to develop nutritional deficiencies. Much of the daily caloric intake of these people is the alcohol they consume, which is deficient in nutritional substances. In addition, alcohol abusers have poor food absorption and increased excretion of nutrients because of diarrhea and fluid loss. When the excessive alcohol consumption stops, the nutritional deficiency can be treated with good food and supplements for a while, if liver disease has not already occurred.

Abuse of other drugs frequently leads to decreased appetite and decreased interest in food. Addicts need supplements of both vitamins and minerals.

People with a chronic wasting illness—This group includes people with malignant disease, chronic malabsorption, hyperthyroidism, chronic obstructive pulmonary disease, congestive heart failure, cystic fibrosis and other illnesses. Nutritional risk is increased because these people have greatly increased caloric and nutritional requirements that are difficult to satisfy with food.

People who have recently undergone surgery—Surgery can cause a relative deficiency, even if a person is well nourished before surgery. People who have undergone surgery on the gastrointestinal tract are particularly likely to develop deficiencies during the post-operative period. Supplementation is very helpful. Vitamins and minerals are frequently administered intravenously until the patient can eat. After that, most people benefit from vitamin and mineral supplements for several weeks after the operation.

People with a portion of the gastrointestinal tract removed—These people are likely to develop deficiencies because important nutrient-absorbing parts of the gastrointestinal tract may be absent from the body. A good multivitamin/mineral preparation usually prevents signs and symptoms of deficiencies. People who have had a significant portion of the stomach removed must take Vitamin B-12 supplements for life (usually by injection).

People who must take medicines—Many medications can cause a deficiency of vitamins and minerals. Specific drugs are listed in the *Interaction with*

Medicine, Vitamins or Minerals section of each chart. For example, laxatives, antacids, medicines to treat epilepsy, and oral contraceptives are a few of the medications that can cause a special need for supplementation of certain vitamins and minerals.

People with recent severe burns or injuries—The nutritional requirements for these people is greatly increased. Adequate supplementation can speed healing and recovery. Ask your doctor for specific advice.

11–Deficiency Symptoms

This section contains a list of proven symptoms of deficiency that have withstood the scrutiny of scientifically controlled studies with results published in medical literature.

12–What this substance does

This section includes a brief discussion of the part each substance plays in chemical reactions or combinations that affect growth, development and health maintenance.

13–Miscellaneous information

Information in this section doesn't fit readily into other information blocks on the charts. For example:

⁂ Cooking tips to preserve the substance during food preparation